A
GOOD
WORD

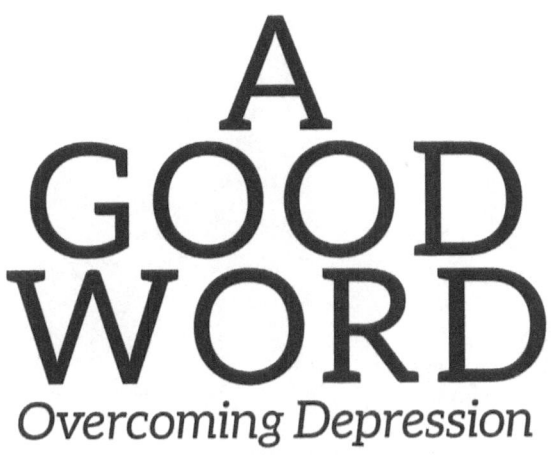

A GOOD WORD

Overcoming Depression

WILLIAM STEWART WHITTEMORE

XULON PRESS

Xulon Press
2301 Lucien Way #415
Maitland, FL 32751
407.339.4217
www.xulonpress.com

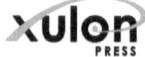

Printed in the United States of America.

ISBN-13:978-1-5456-6169-7

"Anxiety in the heart of man causes depression,
But a good word makes it glad."

Proverbs 12:25 NKJV

Table of Contents

Introduction

Depression is the number one cause of suicide today. Eighty percent of those suffering from depression are not seeking treatment; fifteen percent will commit suicide.

As one who contributed to those statistics, but survived a major suicide attempt, this booklet is offered to help avoid that terrible consequence of not seeking the help that is readily available for combatting depression. In fact, that is the main reason I wrote, "Ransomed: Let the Redeemed of the LORD say so...". It describes the wonderful miracle of my rescue and hopefully it will provide insight to combat this deadly illness too, before one reaches the point of despair I reached.

From my experience I know our Dear Lord is there in all our circumstances to provide that help we need, if only we would call on him. As I experienced, our Lord worked through many fine professionals in bringing the healing I so needed. For example, my psychiatrist treated me for a year then took me off all medication because of the healing work he saw in me. He confided to me one day that he was going to inquire about his patent's faith in the future, apparently because of my dramatic healing. Because of the Lord's intervention, I've been free of all medication for over 25 years now.

Therefore, and hopefully, this information provided in this little booklet will encourage the confidence that our Dear Lord's help is always available to us to overcome depression.

Chapter One

What is Depression?

*"Anxiety in the heart of man causes depression,
But a good word makes it glad."*

Proverbs 12:25 NKJV

Depression is an illness. It is a "whole-body" illness, as defined by the National Institute of Mental Health, involving body, mind and spirit. It affects eating and sleeping, feelings about oneself, and thoughts about things. It affects mood and thoughts. It also attacks the spirit because of the helplessness and hopelessness it sometimes brings. A depressive disorder is not a passing "blue mood." It is not a sign of "personal weakness" or a condition that can be willed or wished away. Anyone with a depressive illness cannot merely "pull themselves together" and get better. Telling someone to "snap out" of a depression makes as much sense as saying to them to "snap out" of diabetes or cancer. Without treatment, symptoms can last for weeks to years and eventually can lead to suicide. Appropriate treatment, however, can help over 80% of those who suffer from depression.

Some Facts About Depression:

Depression is <u>not</u> a personal weakness (54% believe it is).

It is estimated that almost every family in America has been touched in some way by depression (nearly 19 million Americans a year are affected-9.5% of our adult population over age 18); 80% are not having treatment.

By 2020 depression will be the second highest health problem in the world, right behind heart disease.

Major depressive disorder is the #1 cause of disability in the U.S. for ages 15-44.

Suicide is the number 7 to 10 killer in America today (15% of depressed people will commit suicide).

Suicide is the number 2 or 3 killer among our young people. (15-26).

(Note: Research, by Specialty Research Associates, from data supplied by the Department of Health and Human Resources shows that completed youth suicide, among other social ills, "began a dramatic increase after the Engel vs. Vitale Supreme Court decision was made in 1962 which banned school prayer. The rates of youth suicide remained relatively unchanged during the years from 1946 to the School Prayer decision in 1962. But in the years since, suicides among the same group (ages 15-24) have increased 253 percent, or an average of 10.5 percent per year."

1 in 7 teenagers seriously consider suicide.

Preschoolers are the fasted growing market for antidepressants (4%, over a million, are clinically depressed).

Major Categories of Depression:

Bipolar Depression (manic-depressive illness) – A Manic-Depressive illness involves cycles of depression and elation or mania. Sometimes the mood switches are dramatic and rapid, but most often they are gradual. When in the depressed cycle, you can have any or all of the symptoms of a depressive disorder (see symptom list that follows). Mania often affects thinking, judgment, and social behavior in ways that cause serious problems and embarrassment. For example, unwise business or financial decisions may be made when in a manic phase.

Dysthymia Depression - A less severe type of depression, dysthymia involves long-term, chronic symptoms that do not disable, but keep one from functioning at "full steam" or from feeling good. Sometimes people with dysthymia also experience major depressive episodes.

Major Depression – Major Depression is manifested by a combination of symptoms (see symptom list that follows) that interfere with the ability to work, sleep, eat; and enjoy once-pleasurable activities. These disabling episodes of depression can occur once, twice, or several times in a lifetime.

Major Depression is what I suffered leading to my serious suicide attempt.

The key to remember is that, depression is highly treatable by our medical professionals. And most importantly, failure to get treatment for depression can lead to suicide. "Suicide is the most preventable form of death there is" (www.qprinstitute.com).

"God is our refuge and strength, A very present help in trouble."

Psalms 46:1 NKJV

Chapter Two

Causes of Depression

*"The cords of death entangled me,
the anguish of the grave came upon me;
I was overcome by trouble and sorrow."*

Psalms 116:3 NIV

WHAT CAUSES (SOURCE) DEPRESSION?

Physical Ailment (i.e., Hypothyroidism, Concussion, Brain Injury, PTSD, Hypoglycemia)

Unsuccessful Personal Choices (i.e., Drinking, Drugs-my case, Diet)

Severe Emotional Trauma (i.e., Death in the family [especially loss of a parent or child]; Child Abuse, Criticism/Rejection; Violence; Illnesses; Spiritual Crisis)

Sociological Factors (i.e., breakdown of the family structure)

Genetics or Biological (depression tends to run in families)

As one can see, depression is not just a "mental illness". Physical ailments often cause depression. However, in my case, it was wrong personal choices that caused my depression; mainly drinking, and later on, also marijuana. A deadly combination, I believe.

"Where there is no counsel, the people fall;
But in the multitude of counselors there is safety."

Proverbs 11:14 NKJV

Chapter Three

Symptoms of Depression

"My heart is broken. Depression haunts my days".

Job 30:16 TLB

SYMPTOMS OF DEPRESSION

If any of these symptoms are experienced over a continuous two week period, it is imperative that treatment is received immediately:

1) Persistent sad, anxious, or "empty" mood.

2) Feelings of hopelessness, pessimism.

3) Feelings of guilt, worthlessness, helplessness.

4) Loss of interest or pleasure in hobbies and activities. that you once enjoyed.

5) Insomnia, early-morning awakening, or oversleeping.

6) Change in appetite and/or weight loss or overeating and weight gain.

7) Decreased energy, fatigue, being "slowed down".

8) Thoughts of death or suicide, suicide attempts.

9) Restlessness, irritability.

10) Difficulty concentrating, remembering, making decisions or even praying.

11) Persistent physical symptoms that do not respond to treatment, such as headaches, digestive disorders, and chronic pain.

12) Social withdrawal or isolation.

13) Increase in addictive behavior.

14) Lack of Faith, Hope and Love

Note: These are the danger signals for depression. Unfortunately they are not always visible, even to the trained observer.

In my experience with depression I had no trouble in getting to sleep. However, I did not have any dreams, no REM sleep. It was a very black sleep. Also, besides the thoughts of suicide, I was very irritable at times. A family friend told me after my attempt how irritable I was shortly before my attempt. Of course those around me did not know about these symptoms, so they did not realize how in need of help I was in.

And not having a saving relationship with my Lord Jesus Christ, I was without the help I truly needed.

"You, O Lord, keep my lamp burning;
my God turns my darkness into light.".

Psalms 18:28 NIV

Chapter Four

Biblical Experiences of Depression

*"Let the redeemed of the LORD say so,
Whom He has redeemed from the hand of
the enemy,"*

Psalms 107:2 NKJV

One might remember Elijah in 1 Kings 18 having successfully shown the power of God by defeating and executing the prophets of baal. And then forgetting God's power flees in fear from the wrath of Jezebel for what he had done to her prophets.

Therefore in 1 Kings 19:4 we read; *"But he (Elijah) himself went a day's journey into the wilderness, and came and sat down under a broom tree. And he prayed that he might die, and said, "It is enough! Now, Lord, take my life, for I am no better than my fathers!"* However, because of his faith God restored Elijah and gave him a mission to complete for Him (see 1 Kings 19: 5-15). God always has a beautiful purpose for His "fearfully and wonderfully made" sons and daughters (Psalm 139:13-18).

King David was another great servant of the Lord who had his moments of depression, as we can see from Psalm 6:6-7; *"I am weary with my groaning; All night I make my bed swim; I drench my couch with my tears. My eye wastes away because of grief; It grows old because of all my enemies."* However, he most always drew strength from his dependence on the Lord as we see from the end of this classic Psalm in verses 8-10; *"Depart from me, all you workers of iniquity; For the Lord has heard the voice of my weeping. The Lord has heard my supplication; The Lord will receive my prayer. Let all my enemies be ashamed and greatly troubled; Let them turn back and be ashamed suddenly."*

The Apostle Paul suffered much in his ministry proclaiming the Word of God and salvation through Jesus Christ. From beatings to a ship wreck, but he probably hit his lowest point in Asia when he said in 2 Corinthians 1:8,

"For we do not want you to be ignorant, brethren, of our trouble which came to us in Asia: that we were burdened beyond measure, above strength, so that we despaired even of life." However, Paul's faith in our Dear Lord carried him through this difficulty as he states in verse 9;

"Yes, we had the sentence of death in ourselves, that we should not trust in ourselves but in God who raises the dead,". And Jesus will carry us through all our circumstances too. That is the key, trusting in God (Proverbs 3:5-6).

Even Jesus experienced depression. And we can see this when He came into the Garden of Gethsemane to pray;

"And He took with Him Peter and the two sons of Zebedee, and He began to be sorrowful and deeply distressed. Then He said to them, 'My soul is exceedingly sorrowful, even to death. Stay here and watch with Me.'"

Matthew 26:37-38 NKJV

Again, all these encounters with depression show us that traumatic experiences can bring on symptoms of depression, but our faith in the Lord can lead us to the help that we need for overcoming depression. We will cover this more fully in our next chapter.

"Trust in the Lord with all your heart,
And lean not on your own understanding;
In all your ways acknowledge Him,
And He shall direct your paths."

Proverbs 3:5-6 NKJV

Chapter Five

A Good Word in Overcoming Depression

*"Cast your burden on the LORD,
And He shall sustain you;
He shall never permit the righteous to
be moved."*

Psalms 55:22 NKJV

What We Can Do To Overcome Depression

In combatting depression it is very important that we keep certain priorities in life so that the difficulties in life don't side track us. The thoughts, feelings and emotions we have in traumatic experiences are normal in those situations. However, we cannot let them control our actions. Therefore, I have found these five priorities have helped me through many challenging times since my recovery.

I like to call these priorities the "five smooth stones". If you remember in the story of David and Goliath in 1 Samuel 17:40-50, David took "five smooth stones" in his pouch before he faced Goliath in battle. It only took his first stone to slay the giant and so too with our first stone it is the most important of the five. It is Faith.

- Faith – Accepting Jesus Christ as our Lord and Savior; "the way, the truth, and the life" (John 14:6) must be our first priority. And as Jesus also said in Matthew 6:33-34; "But seek first the kingdom of God and His righteousness, and all these things (our needs) shall be added to you. Therefore do not worry about tomorrow, for tomorrow will worry about its own things. Sufficient for the day is its own trouble"; so take one day at a time.

- Family – It is through our family structure we learn about relationships. After God created Adam and Eve He said in Genesis 2:24; "Therefore a man shall leave his father and mother and be joined to his wife, and they shall become one flesh." This is the perfect model for the relationship God wants to have with us; "that they all may be one, as You, Father, are in Me, and I in You; that they also may be one in Us, that the world may believe that You sent Me" (John 17:21).

- Friends – Jesus had close friends in Peter, James and John." Now after six days Jesus took Peter, James, and John his brother, led them up on a high mountain by themselves;" (Matthew 17:1). We need that companionship so we can hold each other up; "Two are better than one, Because they have a good reward for their labor. For if they fall, one will lift up his companion. But woe to him who is alone when he falls, For he has no one to help him up" (Ecclesiastes 4:9-10). Note that these first three deal with others first (Job 42:10).

- Fitness – We need to take care of our bodies they are the only ones we will have in this life. As Paul says in 1 Corinthians 6:19; "Or do you not know that your body is the temple of the Holy Spirit who is in you, whom you have from God, and you

are not your own?" Prayer, a healthy diet
and exercise must be a part of that care,
along with volunteering, which was most
beneficial to my recovery.

• Stewardship – We need to be good stewards of the resources God gives us and
remember our brothers, sisters and the
church in need; "As each one has received
a gift, minister it to one another, as good
stewards of the manifold grace of God"
(1 Peter 4:10).

Going through difficult times is never easy. Again, all
those thoughts, feelings and emotions are normal
in abnormal situations. However, it is very important
to not let them govern our behavior. That's when we
need help, starting with our Lord God, and who He
may bring into the circumstances to walk with us
through them and maintain these priorities.

"Pleasant words are like a honeycomb,
Sweetness to the soul and health
to the bones."

Proverbs 16:24 NKJV

About The Author

William Stewart Whittemore is a blessed father and grandfather. He is a Navy Veteran. Stewart is an experienced hospital chaplain and holds an Advanced Diploma in Lay Biblical Counseling. He looks forward to sharing the Lord's Good Word on overcoming depression and teaching suicide prevention. Stewart has also written and published two books through Xulon Press; "Ransomed: Let the Redeemed of the LORD say so..." and, "But Who Do You Say That I Am?".

Stewart may be contacted through Xulon Press or at: stewart33@earthlink.net

Endorsements

I am grateful to recommend the wide distribution and careful reading of A Good Word; Overcoming Depression by William Stewart Whittemore.

The fourteen pages are informative, medically sound and offers hope to many who will take the information seriously and heed suggested Word in Overcoming Depression. The first and most important of the five priorities relates to Jesus Christ the great physician, healer and restorer of depression and all other mental health disturbances.

George A. Hurst, MD, FACP, FCCP.

I highly recommend this short pamphlet which deals with depression from a biblical point of view. It is very personal and honest from a man who has "been there-done that". Stewart is a godly man who desires that no one else ever have to travel the path that he chose. God has spared his life for the glorious purpose of ministering to the hurting body of Christ and those in need outside the church.

Use this with confidence to reach a person in deep need.

Dr. John Meyer
Pastor of Fellowship Bible Church Venice, FL
Author of the Bible Series:
"Lessons for Life" with 14 titles

"Romans: Our Righteous God Revealed" published by Xulon Press.

Stewart's new book "A Good Word, Overcoming Depression" is a must read for millions of us who suffer depression.

Stewart's crisis' led him to search for the tools necessary to overcome disabling depression and then his heart led him to share the answers he found for the overwhelming pain he tried to escape.

As a combat veteran, life challenges me with many negative emotions, anger, guilt, frustration and depression which easily arise from the unfairness and injustices I experienced as a point man in Vietnam. Stewart's research and observations are a tool that clearly help identify the problems and physical/spiritual healing available to all.

I strongly recommend "A Good Word" to all who may feel overwhelmed at times or who want to help a friend or family member see the treatability of depression.

Dave Wright,
Vietnam Veteran and Author of
"Not Enough Tears"

This simple and heartfelt message can be a life saver for the increasing number of people suffering from depression. The "five smooth stones" offer a practical approach to help one find hope as they redirect their lives. We offer this booklet as a valuable resource at the chapel of our local hospital, where many have picked up a copy for themselves or for a loved one. We are grateful to Stu for this life changing message.

Sandi Richard, M.Div.,
BCC Hospital Chaplain